Instant Pot Vegan Cookbook

10-Ingredients Recipes To Help You Save Time & Money

By

LISA HYDE

Table of Contents

Introduction

Most of us don't have the time, money or luxury to cook meals like mom used to. Instead words like fast, cheap and microwavable have become synonymous with modern eating. To make matters worse, our modern life is often characterized by busy work life demands.

But there is a better way!

In this cookbook, using less than 10 main ingredients, you can cook simple, delicious, healthy meals on a budget and in the smallest of spaces using your handy Instant Pot.

Research has shown that people who cook at home consume less: calories, carbohydrates, sugar, salt and fat than those who cook less or not at all. In short, you can now enjoy all the health benefits with the time-saving 10-ingredients recipes in this cookbook.

Whether you're a beginner or experienced cook, you'll benefit from the easy to follow recipes which have allowed me and others to cook delicious and healthy meals without spending too much time and effort slaving in the kitchen.

If you follow the steps in this cookbook, you'll cook smart and not hard. Others will be wondering how it's possible to get so much done in so little time. As a bonus you'll end up having more time and energy to focus on what is truly important to you while enjoying delicious wholesome meals.

Take action now and transform your Instant Pot into your best kitchen helper ever!

Scroll up to the top and Click Buy Now.

Chapter 1

Veganism In A Nutshell

Veganism has already been hailed as a radical dietary way of life; everyday, more and more people are moving towards eating less meat and more plant-based food. The need to lead a healthy lifestyle in today's modern society is self-evident. More than ever before, we are fighting against environmental pollutants, chemicals, and harmful toxins that undermine our body's immune systems. Eating a nutrient rich healthy diet is no longer a choice for us. Therefore, it makes sense to increase natural and easily digestible foods in our diets to give our body the best chance to lead a completely healthy lifestyle.

Are you tired of spending hours preparing healthy, delicious meals at home? The Instant Pot is the modern kitchen solution to your problem. One great advantage of using Instant Pot is that meals can be cooked quickly. All you need to do is pour in the ingredients, press a few buttons, and let the machine do the rest. There's no need to invest long hours in the kitchen watching over the pot. With Instant Pot, you can prepare fresh, hot, healthy, and nutritious meals everyday in real quick time.

There are multiple benefits of making use of an Instant Pot. Instant Pot is quite easy to operate and clean; it is healthier than any other cooking method and uses pressurized steam for cooking. Its tightly sealed container also prevents essential nutrients from slipping through.

There are endless reasons to add vegan foods in your diet on a daily basis. Vegan recipes are very easy to prepare using an Instant Pot and it allows you to experiment with your favorite ingredients to add your special touch to them.

In this vegan Instant Pot cookbook, you will not only find an exclusive collection of vegan recipes, but you will find diverse cuisines to prepare from your favorite ingredients including breakfasts, snacks, sides, soups, desserts as well as main course meals.

So, what are we waiting for? Let's get started with some nutritious vegan recipes and explore a revolutionary way of preparing vegan cuisines.

Chapter 2

A Revolutionary Vegan Lifestyle

A vegan diet can include vegetables, seeds, nuts, fruits, beans, and pulses. The number of combinations you can create from vegan foods is endless. True veganism is a dietary lifestyle where no animal products are used in preparing recipes. The increasing popularity of vegan diets has a close connection to a growing number of significant and well-documented health benefits.

Whether you go meatless for one day, one month, one year or lifetime, with every day of vegan lifestyle, you will feel better, have more energy and be more resistant to health disorders. It is essential to bear in mind that what you put into your body should be working with your body, rather than against it. It is the same as running uphill as opposed to running along a path. Our body utilizes more energy by digesting meat and processed food as compared to eating easily digested and nutritious vegan foods.

Western civilization consumes a lot more meat than Eastern civilizations. Growth hormones in poultry, milk and other meats are added to increase the growth cycle, and these hormones and pollutants enter your body and carry on their work. This creates many unwanted medical illnesses such as premature puberty, digestive disorders, and asthma.

In order to maintain natural and healthy body growth, you do not need to add growth hormones in your food; all it takes is simply adding more vegetables to your diet. The more natural ingredients you consume, the more you are working towards a better and healthier you.

Nutrient Rich Vegan Diet

Vegan foods are nutrient rich and take care of your body's everyday nutritional needs.

Calcium

- Dark leafy greens, nuts and seeds, fresh and dried fruits & whole wheat bread

Protein

- Seeds, cereals, nuts, grains, beans, & soy/soy products

Vitamins

- Carrots, lettuce, paprika, sweet potato, mangoes, kale, & dried apricots

Potassium

- Potatoes (including the skin), apricots, white beans, yoghurt, & bananas

Iron

- Whole meal/whole wheat/mixed grain bread, grains, leafy greens, tofu, lentils & legumes

Magnesium

- Pumpkin seeds, brown rice, leafy greens & dark chocolate

Vitamin C

- Yellow bell peppers, kiwis, citrus, broccoli, strawberries, & tomatoes

Chapter 3

Instant Pot for Your Wellness & Fitness

Apart from being a revolutionary invention, Instant Pot is also a good investment and quite a helpful kitchen buddy. You can also cook food in batches, freeze them, and then simply heat it up later.

Cooking vegan food has never been easier. You simply need to place all the ingredients into the pot and your job is done. It makes use of pressured steam to help you cook delicious meals. Instant Pot cooking helps in sealing most of the nutrients in the food. Instant Pot is a multi-functional kitchen invention that performs all the functions that you can perform using an electric pressure cooker, a slow cooker, rice cooker, a steamer, and a warming pot.

Why Instant Pot Is the Best For You?

Now that you know the hidden mechanism that is followed by the cooking pot, it is time that you know about some of the core benefits of using an Instant Pot!

Cooking Convenience

An Instant Pot has 12-key functions, which include meat/ stew, soup mode, poultry, rice, bean/chili, multi-grain, steam, porridges, and other control keys.

Each mode has specifications for pressure and time, which can be adjusted as needed.

Saves Time & Energy

Instant Pot takes less time to prepare food as compared to other cooking methods. Instant Pot works particularly well with dried ingredients including beans, grains, legumes, and/or pulses. Instead of pre-soaking them for 2 to 12 hours prior to cooking, you can directly add them into the pot, along with the recommended amount of liquids. At high pressure, you can cook them in less than 30 minutes.

Keeping Nutrients Intact

Unlike many other cooking techniques, which require you to fully immerse the vegetables and other ingredients under the water to cook them, Instant Pot needs just enough water to maintain the steam levels. This technique prevents essential ingredients from being washed away.

Kills off harmful Micro-Organisms

In Instant Pot, the water level is heated to a high temperature where most of the harmful micro-organisms are killed off. It kills harmful bacteria and fungus from grains and vegetables to serve you with healthy meals every time you cook with an Instant Pot.

Chapter 4:

Nutritious Instant Pot Breakfasts

"Eat breakfast like a king, lunch like a prince and dinner like a pauper."

Shake up your wake up with wholesome breakfast recipes. Yum!

1) Classic Blueberry Oats

Prep Time: 5-10 min.

Serves: 1-2

Approx. Calories (per serving): 112

Ingredients:

- 1/2 cup blueberries
- 1 teaspoon chia seeds
- 1/2 cup old fashioned oats
- 1/2 cup almond milk, unsweetened
- Sweetener to taste
- Splash of vanilla
- Pinch of salt
- A pinch of cinnamon
- 1 ½ cups water

Directions:

Pour the water into your Instant Pot and set it aside. In a bowl of medium size, thoroughly mix the mentioned ingredients.

Transfer the bowl mixture to a pint size jar and cover with aluminum foil.

Place the jar on the steamer rack and place them carefully in your Instant Pot.

Cover it and close the pressure vent.

Press "Manual" setting option and set cooking time to 6 minutes. Once the cooking time is done, release the pressure naturally.

Remove the lid and take out the jar. Mix in the oatmeal and serve warm!

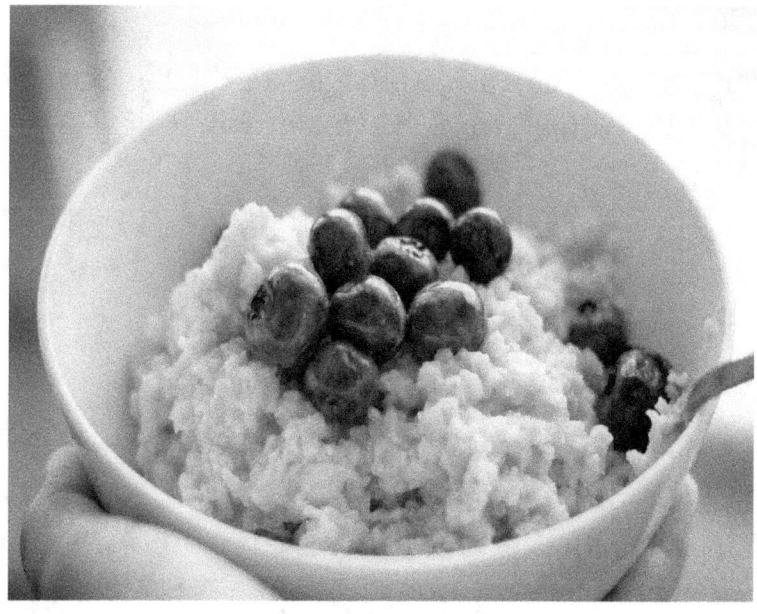

2) Apple Spiced Quinoa

Prep Time: 20-25 min.

Serves: 4

Approx. Calories (per serving): 118

Ingredients:

- ½ cup peeled & diced apple
- ½ cup soy milk
- ½ cup apple, peeled & sliced ½-inch thick
- ¼ cup brown sugar
- ¼ teaspoon cinnamon powder
- 2 cups water
- 1 cup brown or red quinoa, rinsed & drained
- ¼ teaspoon squeezed lemon juice

Directions:

In a bowl of medium size, add the apples and top with the lemon juice. Set aside and drain before using.

Except for garnishes and milk, one by one add the remaining ingredients in your Instant Pot. Close lid, lock, and seal valve.

Cover it and close the pressure vent.

Press "Manual" setting option and set cooking time to 1 minute.

Once the cooking time is done, release the pressure naturally.

Turn off the Instant Pot and open the lid; pour in the milk and season as needed. Spoon equal portions of quinoa into serving bowls.

Garnish with a few slices of apples. Allow to cool before serving.

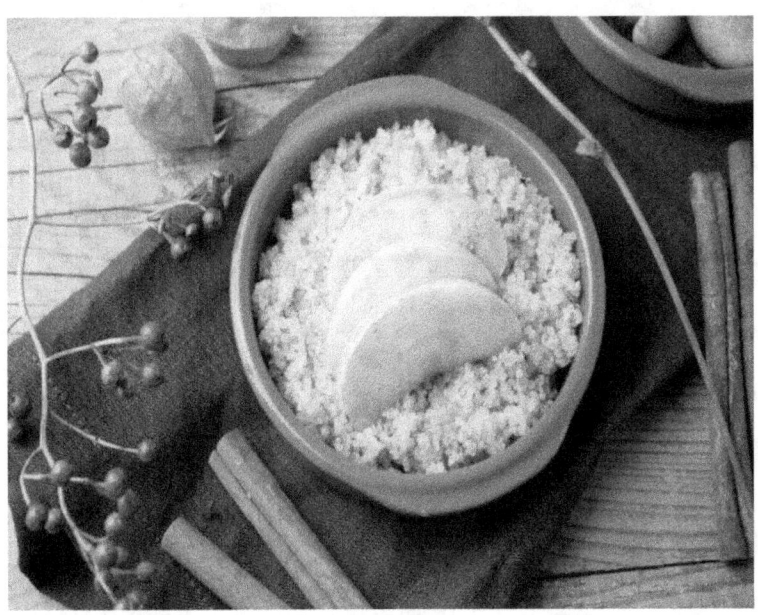

3) Buckwheat Cinnamon Porridge

Prep Time: 15-20 min.

Serves: 2-3

Approx. Calories (per serving): 214

Ingredients:

- 1 ½ cups rice milk
- ½ teaspoon ground cinnamon
- 2 tablespoons raisins
- 2 tablespoons almonds
- 2 tablespoons walnuts
- ¼ teaspoon vanilla
- ½ cup buckwheat ground oats, rinsed
- 1 small banana, sliced

Directions:

At first, take your Instant Pot and one by one add in the mentioned ingredients (reserve the nuts). Stir the ingredients well.

Cover it and close the pressure vent.

Press "Manual" setting option and set cooking time to 6 minutes.

Once the cooking time is done, release the pressure naturally. Add more rice milk if needed.

Serve in bowls; top with the chopped almonds and walnuts.

4) Healthy Peach Oatmeal

Prep Time: 15-20 min.

Serves: 2-3

Approx. Calories (per serving): 186

Ingredients:

- 2 cups water
- 2 peaches, diced
- 1 cup oats
- 1 cup coconut milk

Directions:

In a bowl of medium size, thoroughly mix the ingredients and add the mixture into your Instant Pot.

Cover it and close the pressure vent.

Press "Manual" setting option and set cooking time to 10 minutes. Once the cooking time is done, release the pressure naturally.

Sweeten as desired and serve warm!

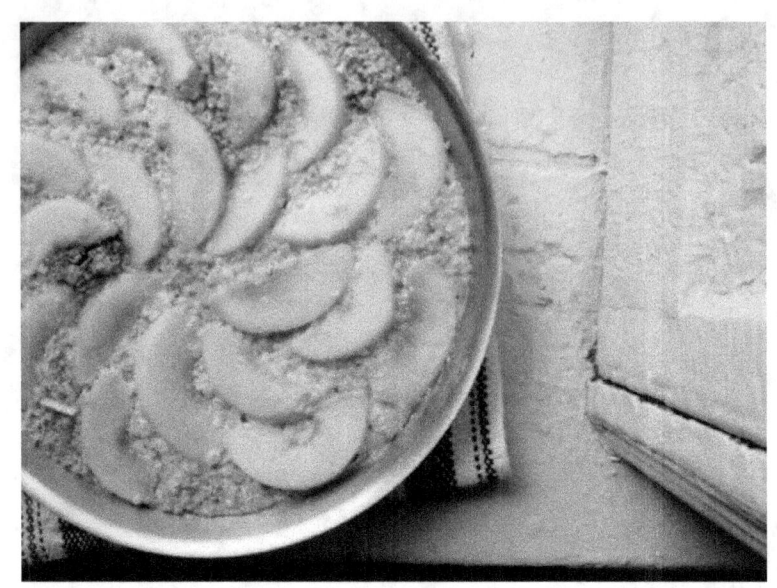

5) Quinoa Corn Morning

Prep Time: 20 min.

Serves: 3-4

Approx. Calories (per serving): 258

Ingredients:

- 1 cup quinoa, do not rinse
- 1 cup water
- 1 can 15 ounces whole corn kernels, rinsed, drained
- ¼ cup chives, minced
- 2 tablespoon olive oil
- 1½ cups mushroom
- 1½ cups vegetable broth, unsalted
- a pinch of white pepper and kosher salt

Directions:

At first, take your Instant Pot and press "Sauté" setting option and add the oil; heat the oil.

Stir-fry the quinoa until it releases a nutty aroma. Add in remaining ingredients in the pot (except chives).

Cover it and close the pressure vent.

Press "Manual" setting option and set cooking time to 1 minute. Once the cooking time is done, release the pressure naturally.

Add equal portions into bowls. Garnish with chives and serve!

6) Millet Cardamom Pilaf

Prep Time: 8-10 min.

Serves: 2-3

Approx. Calories (per serving): 317

Ingredients:

- 1 large onion, sliced
- 2 teaspoons whole cumin
- 1 stick cinnamon
- 2 pods cardamom
- 1 cup decorticated millet
- 1 ½ cups water
- 1 tablespoon oil
- 1 bay leaf
- Salt as required

Directions:

At first, take your Instant Pot and press "Sauté" setting option. Add the oil; heat the oil and then add the whole spices.

Cook until the cumin crackles and then add the onions. Sauté until completely softened.

Turn off the pot and add the millet; sauté until well coated. Pour in the water and salt.

Cover and close the pressure vent.

Press "Manual" setting option and set cooking time to 1 minute. Once the cooking time is done, release the pressure naturally.

Fluff with a fork and serve warm!

7) Carrot Zucchini Mixed Spice Oatmeal

Prep Time: 10-15 min.

Serves: 4-5

Approx. Calories (per serving): 384

Ingredients:

- ½ cup pecans, chopped
- 1/8 teaspoon cloves, ground
- 3/4 teaspoon cinnamon, ground
- 2 teaspoons vanilla extract
- 1/8 teaspoon nutmeg, ground
- 1 small zucchini, peeled, grated
- 1 large carrot, peeled, grated
- 1 cup steel cut oats
- 3 cups vanilla flavored almond milk or soy milk
- 4 tablespoons maple syrup

Directions:

At first, take your Instant Pot and one by one add in the mentioned ingredients. Stir the ingredients well.

Cover and close the pressure vent.

Press "Slow cook" setting option and set cooking time to 3 hours. Serve warm!

8) Cinnamon Hot Chocolate

Prep Time: 10-15 min.

Serves: 8-10

Approx. Calories (per serving): 504

Ingredients:

- 1/8 teaspoon cinnamon, ground
- A pinch salt
- 2/3 cup sugar or to taste
- 8 cups coconut or almond milk, unsweetened
- 2/3 cup cocoa powder
- Coconut whipped cream to serve (optional)

Directions:

At first, take your Instant Pot and one by one add in the mentioned ingredients. Stir the ingredients.

Cover and close the pressure vent.

Press "Slow cook" setting option and set cooking time to 2 hours.

Pour the hot chocolate into mugs. Serve hot with coconut whipped cream on top (optional). Enjoy warm!

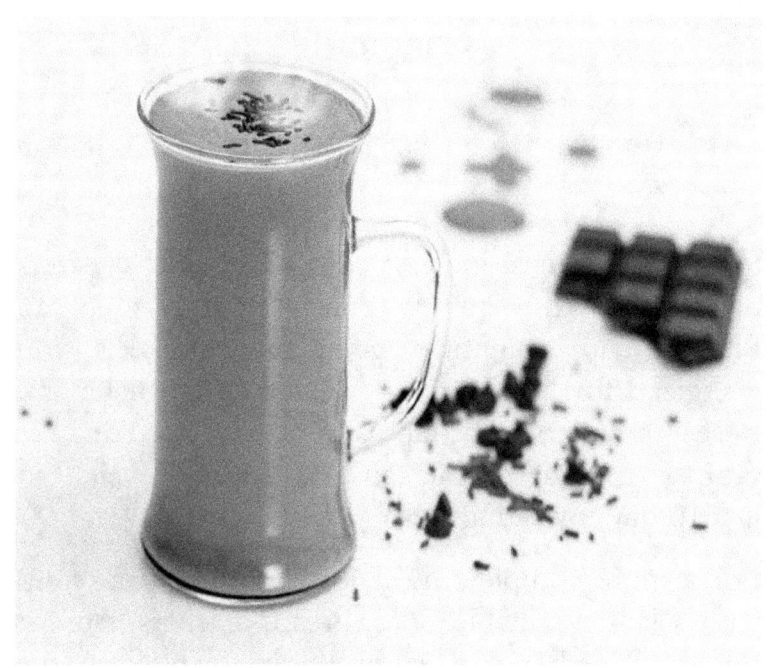

Chapter 5

Mesmerizing Instant Pot Soups & Curry

Soups are a quick and hot comfort meal that offers plenty of health benefits. A tasty bowl of soup can fill you up, minimize cravings and keep you energized for hours with its all-round nourishment. Research has touted soup as a miracle in a bowl for fat loss, as some people can lose stubborn weight in just 10-days by eating soup.

For a more complete meal, you can pair your soup with salads, vegetable sides, bread, crackers, taco or potato. Whether you eat it on its own or at the beginning of your meal -you only need to throw a few ingredients into your Instant Pot to enjoy a bowl of soup in no time!

1) Zucchini Garlic Soup

Prep Time: 30 min.

Serves: 6-8

Approx. Calories (per serving): 102

Ingredients:

- 6 cups vegetable stock
- ½ cup coconut milk
- 1 tablespoon coconut oil or ghee
- 4 cloves garlic, sliced

- 5 medium zucchinis, make small chunks
- 2 onions, quartered
- Ground black pepper and salt to taste

Directions:

At first, take your Instant Pot and press "Sauté" setting option and add the oil, onions, zucchini and garlic; cook for 4-5 minutes. Sauté until completely softened.

Add remaining ingredients except coconut milk.

Cover and close the pressure vent.

Press "Soup" setting option and set cooking time to 15 minutes. Once the cooking time is done, release the pressure naturally.

Add in the coconut milk. Thoroughly blend the mixture with an immersion blender until smooth and serve!

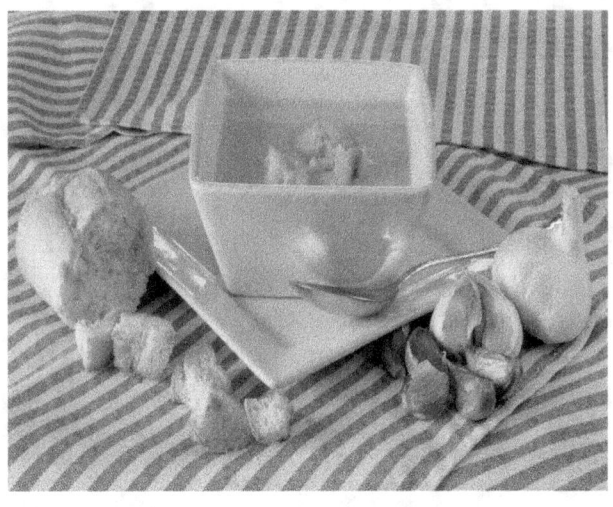

2) Potato Broccoli Soup

Prep Time: 25-30 min.

Serves: 3-4

Approx. Calories (per serving): 234

Ingredients:

- 3 small peeled potatoes, diced
- ½ cup dry lentils, rinsed
- ½ teaspoon garlic powder
- ¼ teaspoon paprika
- 1 medium onion, chopped
- 3 carrots, sliced
- 1 medium head broccoli, make small florets
- 4 cups water
- 1 bay leaf
- ½ teaspoon thyme

Directions:

At first, take your Instant Pot and one by one add in the mentioned ingredients. Season as required and stir them gently.

Cover and close the pressure vent.

Press "Manual" setting option and set cooking time to 15 minutes.

Once the cooking time is done, release the pressure naturally. Discard the bay leaf.

Ladle into soup bowls and serve warm!

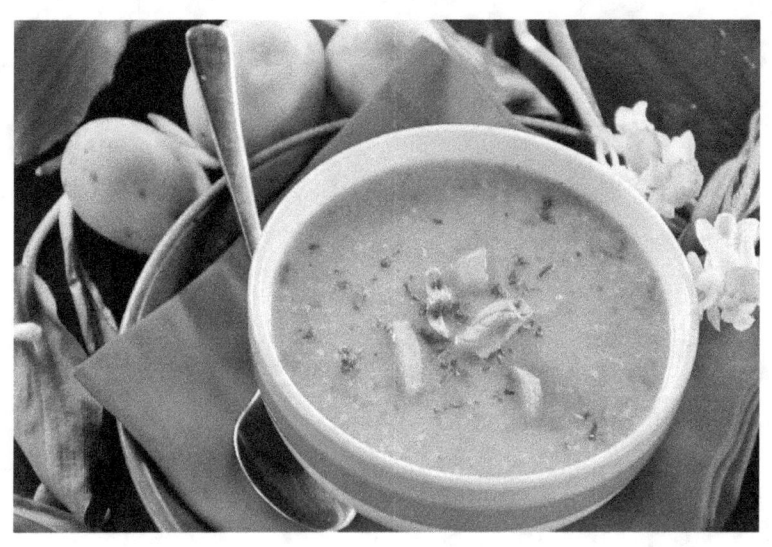

3) Protein Rich Mixed Bean Soup

Prep Time: 10-15 min.

Serves: 4

Approx. Calories (per serving): 357

Ingredients:

- 1 teaspoon onion powder
- 4 ounces diced tomatoes
- 4 ounces kidney beans
- 4 ounces butter beans
- 4 ounces cannellini beans
- 4 ounces refried beans
- 4 ounces black beans
- 4 cloves garlic, minced
- Pepper and salt to taste
- 4 cups water

Directions:

At first, take your Instant Pot and one by one add in the mentioned ingredients. Stir them gently.

Cover and close the pressure vent.

Press "Slow cook" setting option and set cooking time to 2 hours.

Ladle into soup bowls and serve warm!

4) Scrumptious Squash Curry

Prep Time: 30 min.

Serves: 5-6

Approx. Calories (per serving): 88

Ingredients:

- 1 teaspoon curry powder
- 1 (3 pound) peeled butternut squash, diced
- 3 cups water
- 1/2 cup coconut milk
- 1 ½ teaspoon sea salt
- 1 teaspoon olive oil
- 1 chopped onion
- 2 garlic cloves, minced
- Hulled pumpkin seeds & dried cranberries (optional) for toppings

Directions:

At first, take your Instant Pot and press "Sauté" setting option and add the oil and onions; cook for 1 minute. Sauté until completely softened.

Mix in the curry powder and garlic; continue cooking until they are fragrant for 1 more minute.

Switch off the pot and mix in the diced squash. Pour in the water and salt. Cover and close the pressure vent.

Press "Soup" setting option and set cooking time to 10 minutes. Once the cooking time is done, release the pressure naturally.

Remove the lid and use an immersion blender to puree the cooked mixture.

Add the soup to serving bowls and add the coconut milk; adjust the seasoning as needed.

Serve warm and top with the pumpkin seeds and dried cranberries.

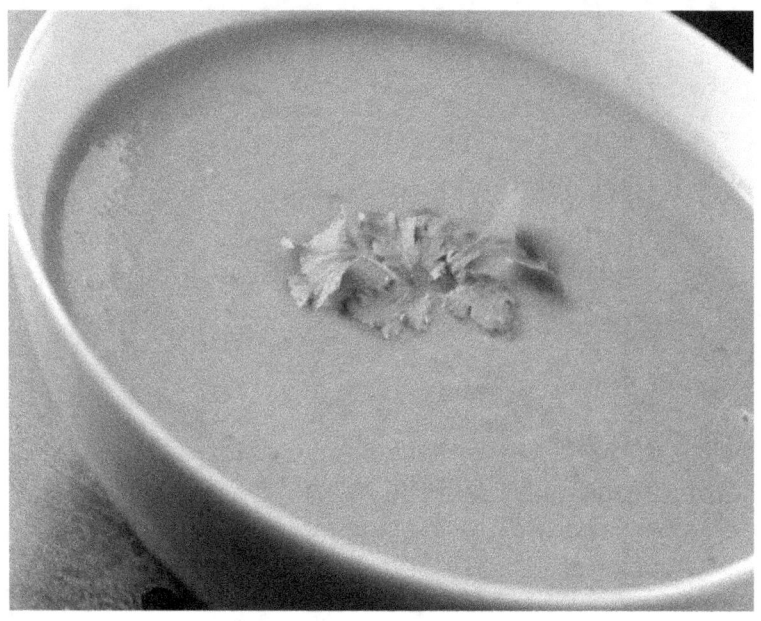

5) Lemongrass Veggie Soup

Prep Time: 25-30 min.

Serves: 6

Approx. Calories (per serving): 286

Ingredients:

- 6 stalks lemongrass, chopped
- 3 cups coconut milk
- juice of one lime
- 4 cloves garlic, pressed
- 1 inch piece of minced ginger
- 2 onions, roughly chopped
- 6 large peeled carrots, roughly chopped
- 2 large zucchinis, roughly chopped
- Fresh cilantro leaves, chopped

Directions:

At first, take your Instant Pot and one by one add in the mentioned ingredients (reserve zucchini).

Pour water to cover the ingredients. Cover and close the pressure vent.

Press "Soup" setting option and set cooking time to 15 minutes. Once the cooking time is done, add the zucchini.

Close the lid. Press "Steam" setting option and set cooking time to 15 minutes. Cool for a while and blend with a stick blender.

Pour into serving bowls and garnish with cilantro. Serve the mixture warm.

6) Potato Cashew Soup

Prep Time: 20-25 min.

Serves: 4-5

Approx. Calories (per serving): 195

Ingredients:

- 1/2 cup onions, chopped
- 3 whole garlic cloves
- 1/2 cup nutritional yeast
- 1 teaspoon turmeric, chopped
- 1/2 cup raw cashews
- 2 cups potatoes, peeled and chopped
- 1 cup carrots, chopped
- 1 teaspoon salt
- 2 cups water

Directions:

At first, take your Instant Pot and one by one add in the mentioned ingredients.

Cover and close the pressure vent.

Press "Manual" setting option and set cooking time to 5 minutes.

Once the cooking time is done, release the pressure naturally.

Remove the lid and transfer the cooked mixture into a food processor, blend to make a creamy and super smooth soup mixture. Serve warm.

Chapter 6

One Pot Lunch & Dinner Meals

Everyone loves one-pot meals because they require little fuss and minimal clean-up. It is simple while offering diversity with multiple ingredients. You can serve your one-pot meal with some warm rolls, naan or tacos on the side. To save time, you can cook double portions and freeze the leftovers for the week.

1) Italian Ricotta Casserole

Prep Time: 20-25 min.

Serves: 10

Approx. Calories (per serving): 314

Ingredients:

For the cashew-tofu ricotta:

- 1 ½ packages (15 ounces each) firm tofu
- 6 cloves garlic
- 1 cup soy milk or almond milk
- 1 cup nutritional yeast
- 1 cup cashews
- Salt to taste
- 4 teaspoons lemon juice (optional)
- Freshly ground black pepper as required

For the casserole:

- 2 large eggplants, thinly sliced
- 2 jars (25 ounces each) marinara sauce

Directions:

Place all the ingredients of the tofu ricotta into a blender and blend to make a smooth mixture. Chill for 4-6 hours.

Now to make the casserole, coat the Instant Pot with a cooking spray.

Add a little of the marinara sauce in the bottom. Top with some eggplant slices. Spread some of the ricotta mixture on top.

Repeat the layers until all the ingredients are used up.

Cover and close the pressure vent. Press "Slow cook" setting option and set cooking time to 2-3 hours.

Once the cooking time is done, release the pressure naturally. Serve warm with cooked pasta.

2) Potato Veggie Curry

Prep Time: 30 min.

Serves: 4

Approx. Calories (per serving): 236

Ingredients:

- 2 onions, chopped
- 3 teaspoons oil
- ¼ cup curry paste, as required
- 2 cans light coconut milk
- 2 cups vegetable stock
- 3 cups button mushrooms
- 2 medium potatoes, peeled and make chunks
- 2 eggplants, make chunks
- 2 tablespoons cilantro
- Salt as required

Directions:

At first, take your Instant Pot and press "Sauté" setting option and add the oil, onions, and potatoes; cook for 2-3 minutes. Sauté until completely softened.

Add eggplant and mushrooms. Stir well and continue cooking for about 4-5 minutes. Pour the paste, stock and coconut milk and stir the mixture.

Press "Cancel"; cover and close the pressure vent.

Press "Manual" setting option and set cooking time to 10 minutes.

Once the cooking time is done, release the pressure naturally. Garnish with cilantro and serve with cooked rice.

3) Nutritious Collard Wraps

Prep Time: 30 min.

Serves: 7-8

Approx. Calories (per serving): 183

Ingredients:

- 1 ¼ cups dry black eyed peas, rinsed
- 6 cloves garlic, minced
- 1 teaspoon thyme, dried
- 4 teaspoons soy sauce
- 1 teaspoon dried basil
- 1 1/3 cups semi pearled farro, soaked in water for 30 minutes
- 1 onion, chopped
- 3 tablespoons olive oil
- 6-8 collard green leaves
- 1 teaspoon hot sauce
- Salt as required
- 2 cups water
- 2 cups broth
- 2 tablespoons oil

Directions:

At first, take your Instant Pot and press "Sauté" setting option and add the oil, and farro; cook for a few minutes.

Add remaining ingredients except broth and collard. Sauté the mixture until well coated. Add the salt and broth. Stir the mixture a little.

Cover and close the pressure vent.

Press "Manual" setting option and set cooking time to 10 minutes. Once the cooking time is done, release the pressure naturally. Serve warm.

Place the collard greens on kitchen platform. Spread the mixture over collard greens, roll and serve.

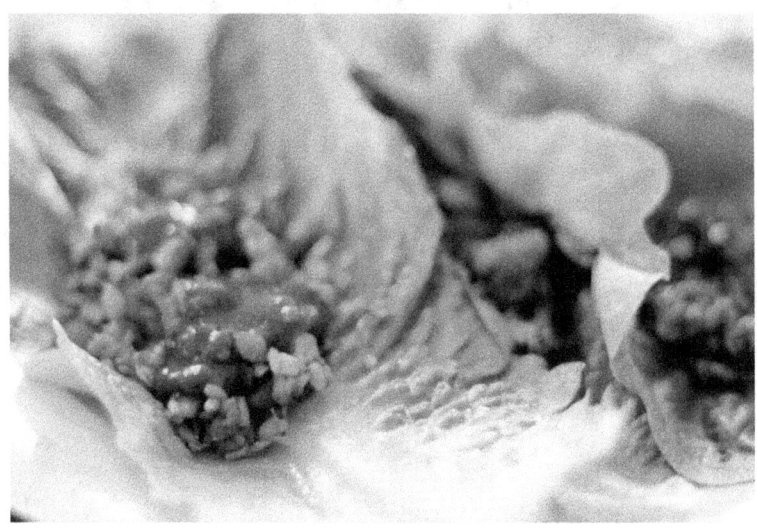

4) Spiced Bean Tacos

Prep Time: 10-15 min.

Serves: 6-8

Approx. Calories (per serving): 592

Ingredients:

- 1 ½ cups corn kernels, fresh or frozen
- 1 ½ cans (6 ounces each) tomato paste
- 1 cup chili sauce
- 1 teaspoon cinnamon, ground
- 1 ½ tablespoons cocoa, unsweetened
- 3 cans (15 ounces each) pinto beans, drained
- 2 chipotle peppers, chopped
- 1 ½ teaspoons ground cumin
- Salt as required

For serving:

- 1 tomato, thinly sliced
- 1 peeled and pitted avocado, make slices
- Taco shells as needed
- 1 cup lettuce, thinly sliced
- 2-3 teaspoons lime juice

Directions:

At first, take your Instant Pot and one by one add in the mentioned ingredients. Stir the ingredients well with each other.

Cover and close the pressure vent.

Press "Slow cook" setting option and set cooking time to 90 minutes.

Once the cooking time is done, release the pressure naturally. Serve warm.

Add the filling in the tacos. Add some lettuce, tomatoes and avocadoes. Sprinkle lime juice over and enjoy!

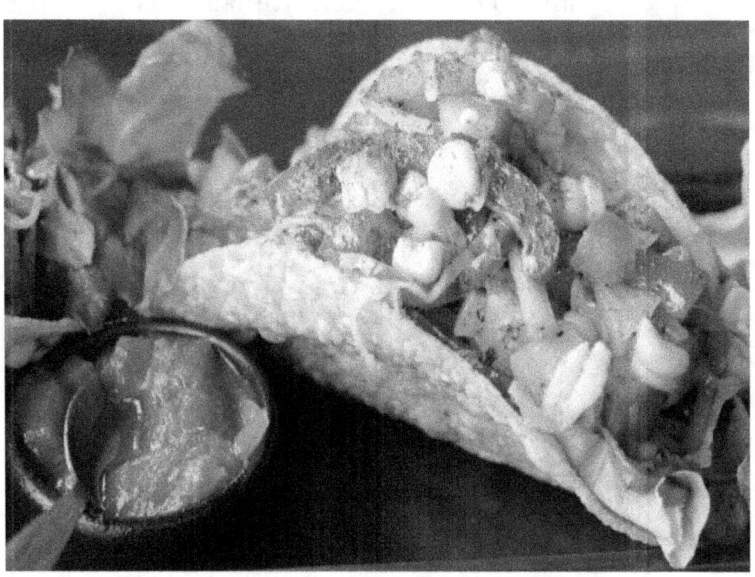

5) Classic Veggie Barley Casserole

Prep Time: 30 min.

Serves: 6

Approx. Calories (per serving): 345

Ingredients:

- 4 cloves garlic, minced
- 2 large carrots, chopped
- 2 cups mushrooms, make slices
- 3 cups vegetable stock
- 4 celery stalks, chopped
- 2 cups pearl barley
- 2 bell peppers, chopped
- 2 onions, chopped
- 3 cups mixed vegetable juice
- ½ cup walnuts, chopped
- Salt as required

Directions:

At first, take your Instant Pot and one by one add in the mentioned ingredients except walnuts. Stir the ingredients well with each other.

Cover and close the pressure vent.

Press "Manual" setting option and set cooking time to 25 minutes.

Once the cooking time is done, release the pressure naturally. Serve warm with walnuts on top.

6) Vegan Potato Meal

Prep Time: 30 min.

Serves: 4-5

Approx. Calories (per serving): 166

Ingredients:

- 4 cloves garlic, make halves
- 1 bay leaf
- 2 tablespoons vegan butter
- 1 can (14 ounce) vegetable broth
- 1 ½ pounds russet potatoes, peeled, make 2 inch pieces
- ½ cup almond milk
- ½ teaspoon salt
- Freshly ground black pepper as required

Directions:

Add the broth, potatoes, garlic and bay leaf to the pot.

Cover and close the pressure vent.

Press "Manual" setting option and set cooking time to 8 minutes. Once the cooking time is done, release the pressure naturally.

Strain the potato mixture. Preserve the strained liquid and remove bay leaf. Transfer the potatoes to the Instant Pot and mash them using a potato masher.

Place a saucepan of medium size over medium heat. Add the milk, salt and butter; melt the butter completely.

Pour the mixture into the pot. Pour the strained liquid.

Cover and close the pressure vent.

Press "Slow cook" setting option and set cooking time to 10-15 minutes. Once the cooking time is done, release the pressure naturally.

Serve warm and sprinkle freshly crushed pepper.

7) Vegan Fried Rice Feast

Prep Time: 15 min.

Serves: 4-5

Approx. Calories (per serving): 614

Ingredients:

- 2 tablespoons olive oil
- ⅓ cup scallions, sliced
- 3 cups multi-grain rice or brown rice, uncooked
- 1 cup carrots, grated
- 1 cup frozen peas
- 3 1/2 cups water
- 2 tablespoons soy sauce

Directions:

At first, take your Instant Pot and one by one add in the mentioned ingredients except peas. Stir the ingredients well with each other.

Cover and close the pressure vent.

Press "Multigrain" setting option and set cooking time to 10 minutes. Once the cooking time is done, release the pressure naturally.

Add the peas and mix well. Serve warm.

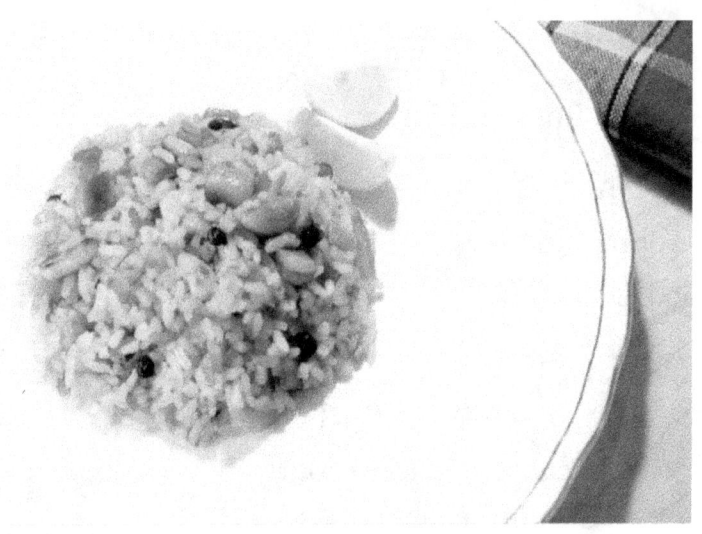

8) Vegan Treat with Grains & Veggies

Prep Time: 20-25 min.

Serves: 3-4

Approx. Calories (per serving): 415

Ingredients:

- 1 tablespoon oil
- 1 large onion, sliced
- 4 cups vegetable broth
- 2 cups mushrooms, sliced
- 1 cup summer squash, make thin slices
- 1 cup green beans, make thin slices
- 1 ¼ cups decorticated organic millet
- 1/ 3 cup green lentils, rinsed, soaked overnight
- ½ cup fresh mixed herbs
- 1 stick cinnamon
- Salt as required
- 2 tablespoons lemon juice
- 4 cloves garlic, sliced

Directions:

At first, take your Instant Pot and press "Sauté" setting option and add the oil, onions, mushroom, and garlic; cook for 4-5 minutes. Sauté until completely softened.

Add the herbs and sauté until fragrant. Add the millet and sauté until well coated. Pour the broth and salt; stir a little.

Cover and close the pressure vent.

Press "Manual" setting option and set cooking time to 10 minutes. Open the lid, add the veggies and stir.

Cover and close the pressure vent. Press "Manual" setting option and set cooking time to 2 minutes.

Once the cooking time is done, release the pressure naturally. Add lemon juice, stir and serve warm.

9) Sprouts & Toasted Peanuts

Prep Time: 25-30 min.

Serves: 4

Approx. Calories (per serving): 796

Ingredients:

- ½ tablespoon palm sugar
- ½ tablespoon peanut oil
- ¼ tsp. fresh lemon zest
- ⅛ cup water
- 3 cups cooked white rice
- 1½ pounds brussels sprout, bottoms trimmed, make large pieces
- ⅛ tsp. kosher salt
- 3 tablespoon lemon juice
- ¼ cup roasted, peanuts

Directions:

At first, take your Instant Pot and one by one add in the mentioned ingredients except lemon juice, peanuts, rice, and salt. Stir the ingredients well with each other.

Cover and close the pressure vent.

Press "Manual" setting option and set cooking time to 4 minutes. Once the cooking time is done, release the pressure naturally.

Open the lid, add the lemon juice, peanuts and salt.

Add equal portions of braised vegetables onto plates; serve with steamed rice on the side.

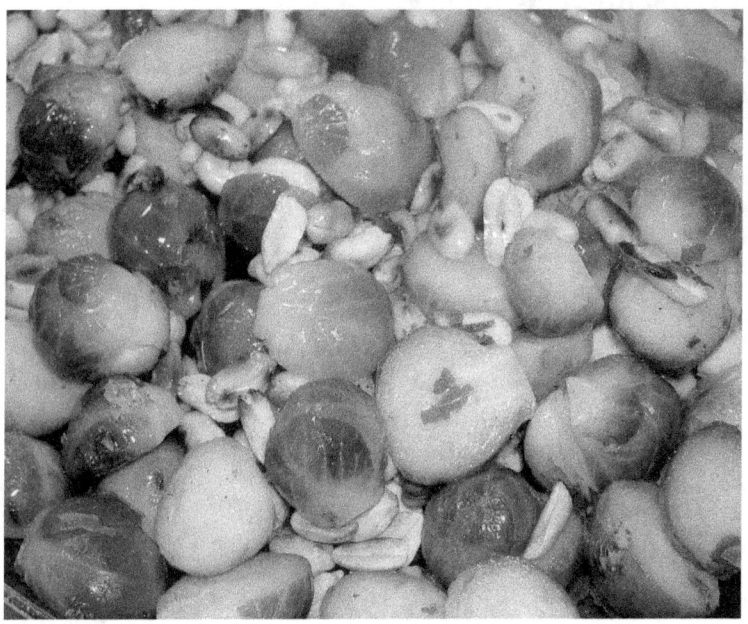

10) Classic Bean & Rice

Prep Time: 25-30 min.

Serves: 4

Approx. Calories (per serving): 345

Ingredients:

- 2 cloves minced garlic
- 1 cup dry black beans, rinsed
- ½ cup onions, chopped
- 4 ½ cups water
- ½ teaspoon salt
- 1 cup brown rice, rinsed
- Avocado slices
- Lime wedges

Directions:

At first, take your Instant Pot and one by one add in the mentioned ingredients. Stir the ingredients well with each other.

Cover and close the pressure vent.

Press "Manual" setting option and set cooking time to 28 minutes. Once the cooking time is done, release the pressure naturally.

Ladle into serving bowls. Squeeze a lime wedge in each bowl and stir. Garnish with avocado slices on top.

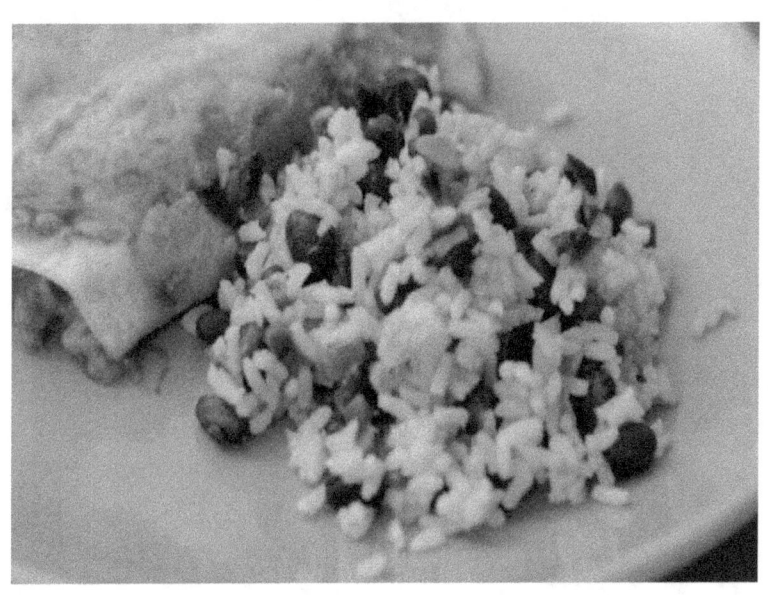

11) Squash Almond Retreat

Prep Time: 25-30 min.

Serves: 4

Approx. Calories (per serving): 532

Ingredients:

- 1 tablespoon olive oil
- 1 cup mushroom and vegetable broth, unsalted
- ½ cup almond slivers, freshly toasted
- ¼ cup minced white onion
- ⅛ cup minced chives
- 1 pound butternut squash, cubed
- 1 pound French beans, ends removed, sliced into 2-inch long slivers
- A pinch of white pepper
- ¼ tsp. kosher salt

Directions:

At first, take your Instant Pot and press "Sauté" setting option and add the oil and onions; cook for 4-5 minutes. Sauté until completely softened.

Except for almonds, chives, and beans, one by one add the ingredients into the pot.

Cover and close the pressure vent.

Press "Manual" setting option and set cooking time to 10 minutes. Once the cooking time is done, release the pressure naturally.

Open the lid, stir in the beans. Secure lid for 2 minutes to warm the beans. Adjust seasoning if needed.

Add equal portions of vegetables into plates. Top with almond slivers and chives; serve.

12) Garlic Lentil Risotto

Prep Time: 25-30 min.

Serves: 5-6

Approx. Calories (per serving): 408

Ingredients:

- 1 large onion, chopped
- 5 cups vegetable broth
- 2 tablespoons parsley, chopped
- 2 celery stalks, chopped
- 5 cloves minced garlic
- 1 ½ cups dry lentils, soaked overnight and drained
- 1 ½ cups Arborio rice
- 1 tablespoon olive oil
- Pepper and salt as required

Directions:

At first, take your Instant Pot and press "Sauté" setting option and add the oil, onions, and garlic; cook for 4-5 minutes. Sauté until completely softened.

Add the rice and cook for a couple of minutes until the rice becomes opaque. Add broth, salt, pepper, celery, and parsley. Combine well.

Press 'Cancel' button. Cover and close the pressure vent.

Press "Manual" setting option and set cooking time to 5 minutes. Once the cooking time is done, release the pressure naturally. Serve warm.

13) Magical Mushroom Risotto

Prep Time: 20-25 min.

Serves: 4

Approx. Calories (per serving): 242

Ingredients:

- 1 teaspoon olive oil
- 1 ½ cups white or cremini mushrooms
- 1 ½ cups chopped portobello mushrooms
- 2 teaspoons vegan butter
- 3 cups vegetable broth
- 1 1/2 cup Arborio rice, uncooked
- 2 cloves minced garlic
- 1 cup white onion, diced
- ½ cup white wine
- 3 teaspoons lemon juice
- Ground pepper and salt as required

Directions:

Take a saucepan of medium size and add in the butter (1 tsp.) and both mushrooms; cook over medium heat.

Cook until soft and tender then set aside.

Take your Instant Pot and press "Sauté" setting option and add the oil, butter (1 tsp.), onion and garlic; cook for 4-5 minutes. Sauté until completely softened.

Add the rice and combine well; cook to make the rice translucent. Add the wine, cooked mushrooms; cook until the wine evaporates.

Pour the stock on top and stir.

Cover and close the pressure vent.

Press "Manual" setting option and set cooking time to 5 minutes. Once the cooking time is done, release the pressure naturally. Serve warm.

Transfer onto a serving plate; add the seasoning and lemon juice.

Serve the risotto warm.

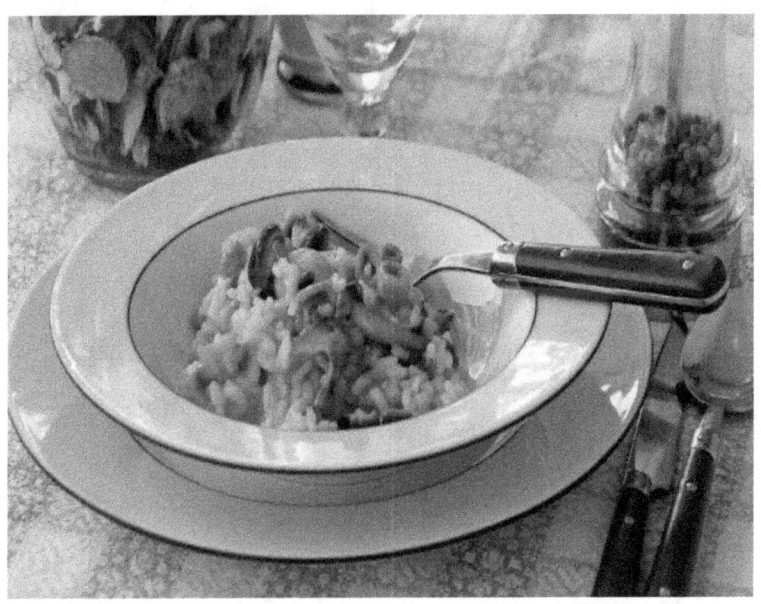

14) Mango Rice Lunch Treat

Prep Time: 20-25 min.

Serves: 2-3

Approx. Calories (per serving): 52

Ingredients:

- 1 cup mango chunks, frozen
- 2 tablespoons brown sugar
- 1 cup white jasmine rice
- 1 ¼ cups light sweetened coconut milk
- Additional 1/3 cup light sweetened coconut milk
- Black sesame seeds

Directions:

Add white jasmine rice (1 cup), mango, and coconut milk (1 ¼ cup) in the pot.

Cover and close the pressure vent.

Press "Manual" setting option and set cooking time to 4 minutes. Once the cooking time is done, release the pressure naturally.

Pour some extra coconut milk (1/3 cup) once done and mix well.

Add the mix into serving bowls and top with brown sugar alongside some sesame seeds. Serve warm.

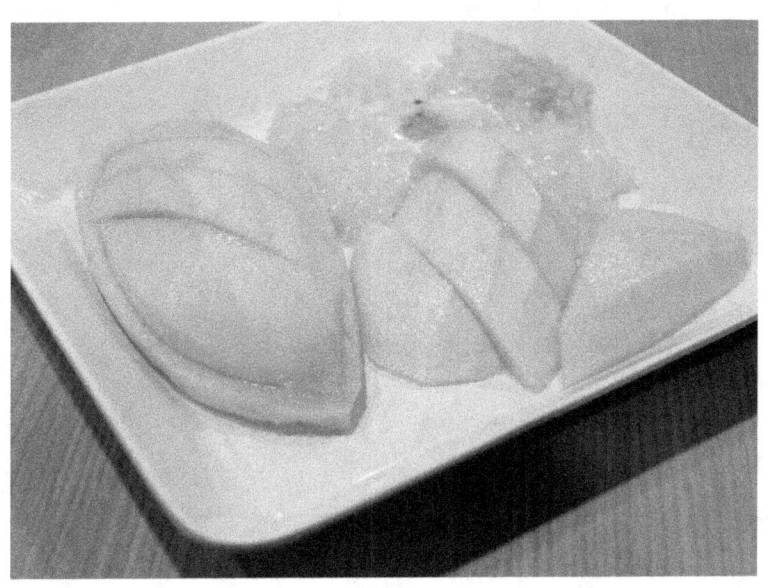

15) Beet Walnut Bowl

Prep Time: 15-20 min.

Serves: 4

Approx. Calories (per serving): 152

Ingredients:

- 1 1/2 pounds beets, scrubbed, rinsed
- 2 cups water

For the dressing:

- 1 1/2 tablespoons extra virgin olive oil
- 2 tablespoons walnuts, finely chopped
- 2 teaspoons lemon juice
- 1 teaspoon Dijon mustard
- 2 teaspoons apple cider vinegar
- 1 1/2 teaspoons sugar
- Pepper and salt as required

Directions:

At first, add beets and water into the pot.

Cover and close the pressure vent.

Press "Manual" setting option and set cooking time to 10 minutes. Once the cooking time is done, release the pressure naturally.

Drain the beets and chop into bite sized pieces and place in a serving bowl.

In a mixing bowl, add all the ingredients of the dressing except oil and walnuts.

Whisk well and add the olive oil slowly into the dressing; combine well. Drizzle the dressing over the beets, toss and serve.

16) Asian Style Quinoa & Veggies

Prep Time: 15-20 min.

Serves: 2-3

Approx. Calories (per serving): 247

Ingredients:

- 2 tablespoons soy sauce
- 2 tablespoons rice vinegar
- 1 thumb grated ginger
- 2 tablespoons of sugar
- 2 cups quinoa
- 4 cups water
- 8-ounce bag mixed vegetables, frozen

Directions:

Thaw the vegetables.

Take your Instant Pot and one by one add in the mentioned ingredients except veggies. Stir the ingredients well with each other.

Cover and close the pressure vent.

Press "Manual" setting option and set cooking time to 1 minute. Once the cooking time is done, release the pressure naturally.

Open up the lid and add in the vegetables; serve warm.

Chapter 7:

Scrumptious Instant Pot Sides & Snacks

1) Instant Pot Golden Fries

Prep Time: 25-30 min.

Serves: 7-8

Approx. Calories (per serving): 78

Ingredients:

- 2 teaspoons kosher salt
- Canola oil to deep fry as needed
- 2 pounds russet potatoes, peeled and sliced to make fries
- 1/2 teaspoon baking soda
- 2 cups cold water

Directions:

At first, take your Instant Pot and one by one add the baking soda, salt and water. Stir the ingredients well with each other. Place a steamer basket inside and add the potatoes without overlapping.

Cover and close the pressure vent.

Press "Manual" setting option and set cooking time to 2 minutes. Once the cooking time is done, release the pressure naturally. Take out the fries.

Take a deep frying pan of medium size and add in the oil to half depth of the pan; heat the pan over medium heat.

Add fries in batches and fry until light golden brown in color.

Place over paper towels and top with salt; serve warm.

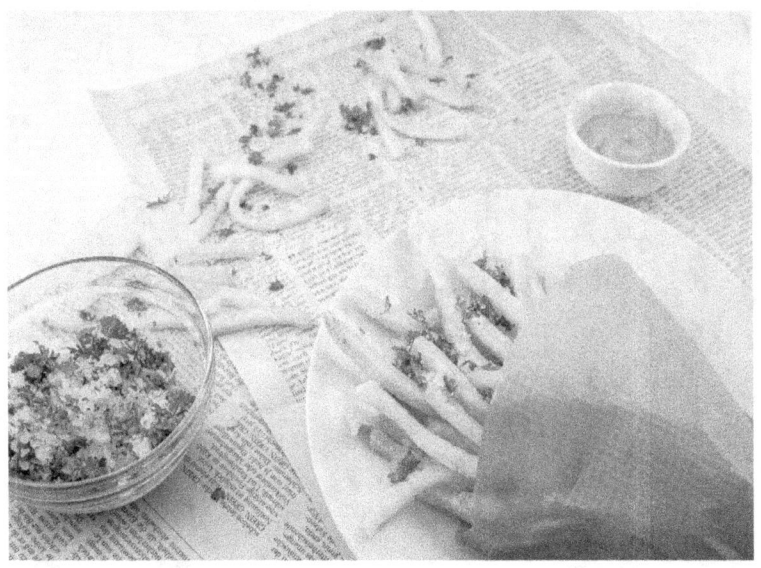

2) Spiced Tofu

Prep Time: 15-20 min.

Serves: 2

Approx. Calories (per serving): 242

Ingredients:

- 1/2 tablespoon red pepper flakes
- 3/4 cup ketchup
- 1/2 tablespoon apple cider vinegar
- 1 tablespoon soy sauce
- 1 container extra firm tofu, make 1 inch cubes
- 1/4 teaspoon garlic powder
- 1/4 teaspoon salt
- 1 1/2 tablespoons brown sugar

Directions:

At first, take your Instant Pot and one by one add in the mentioned ingredients. Stir the ingredients well with each other.

Cover and close the pressure vent.

Press "Slow cook" setting option and set cooking time to 2 ½ hours. Once the cooking time is done, release the pressure naturally.

If there is too much liquid, simmer until dry. Stir and serve warm.

3) Yummy Lemon Corn

Prep Time: 20-25 min.

Serves: 5-6

Approx. Calories (per serving): 132

Ingredients:

- 6 ears corn, remove the husk
- Seasoning (spice mixture) of your choice
- Lemon juice (optional)

Directions:

At first, take your Instant Pot and add the corn in the steamer. Stir the ingredients well with each other.

Cover and close the pressure vent.

Press "Manual" setting option and set cooking time to 15 minutes. Once the cooking time is done, release the pressure naturally.

Sprinkle a seasoning of your choice and brush with lemon juice.

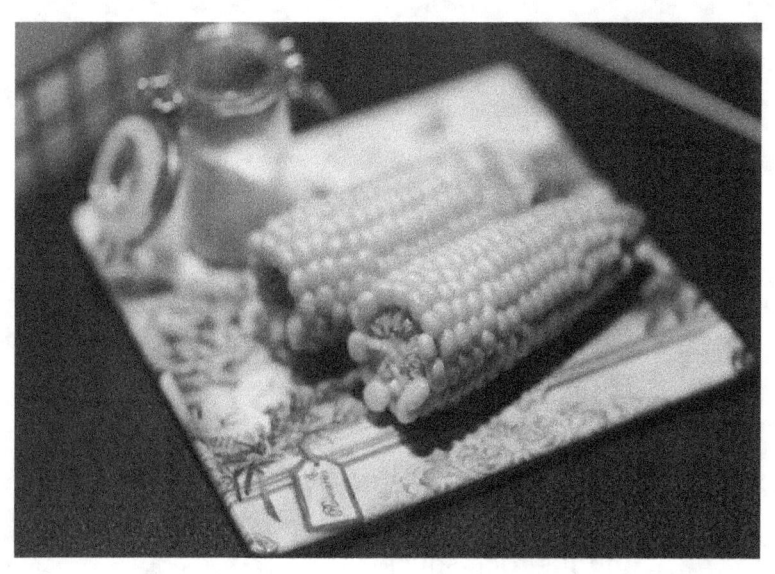

4) Cinnamon & Pepper Peanuts

Prep Time: 30 min.

Serves: 7-8

Approx. Calories (per serving): 643

Ingredients:

- 4 star anise
- 6 cloves garlic
- 2 pounds raw peanuts, large size and with shell
- 2 chunks rock sugar
- 4 sticks cinnamon
- 8 red chili peppers, dried (optional)

Directions:

At first, take your Instant Pot and one by one add in the mentioned ingredients. Stir the ingredients well with each other. Pour enough water to cover the peanuts.

Cover and close the pressure vent.

Press "Manual" setting option and set cooking time to 25 minutes. Once the cooking time is done, release the pressure naturally.

Shell peanuts and serve warm.

5) Eggplant Chickpea Hummus

Prep Time: 15 min.

Serves: 6-7

Approx. Calories (per serving): 139

Ingredients:

- 2 cloves garlic, peeled
- 1/4 teaspoon paprika
- 1/4 teaspoon smoked paprika
- 1 cup water
- 2 tablespoons lemon juice
- 2 pound eggplant, peeled, make quarters lengthwise
- 3/4 cup cooked chickpeas
- 2 tablespoons tahini
- 1/4 teaspoon ground cumin
- 1 teaspoon salt
- 1/4 teaspoon sumac to garnish

Directions:

Pour water in your Instant Pot. Place a steamer basket and arrange the eggplant quarters.

Cover and close the pressure vent.

Press "Manual" setting option and set cooking time to 3 minutes. Once the cooking time is done, release the pressure naturally.

Place the eggplant into a blender. Add the garlic and blend until smooth.

Add the tahini, chickpeas, both types of paprika, cumin, salt and lemon juice and blend again until well combined. Sprinkle sumac and serve in bowls.

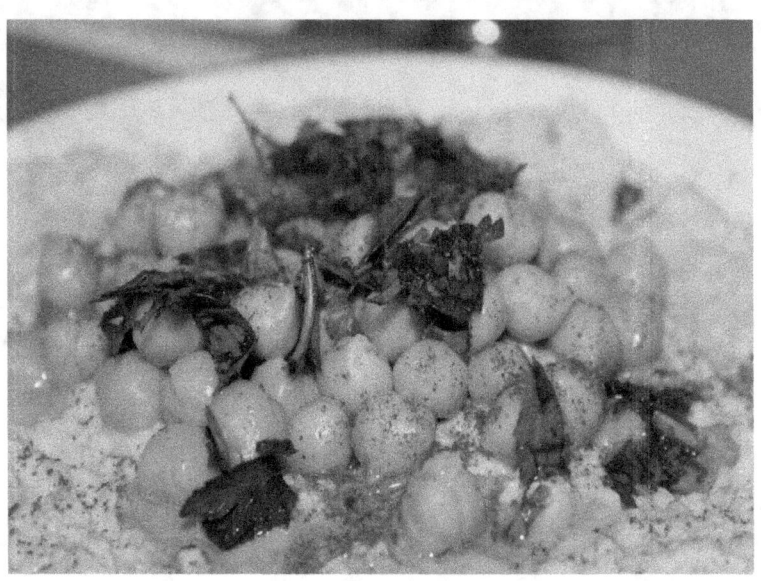

Chapter 8:

Delicious Instant Pot Desserts

Do you know the right indulgences can fuel your mind and body? When we approach desserts the right way, they can improve our emotional and physical wellness. Research has shown that dieters who paid attention and savored every bite of their desserts lost and kept their weight-loss compared to dieters who restricted themselves.

So have your cake and eat it too but savor mindfully!

1) Classic Rice Cinnamon Pudding

Prep Time: 25-30 min.

Serves: 4

Approx. Calories (per serving): 362

Ingredients:

- 1 cup rinsed jasmine rice, drained
- ¼ cup brown sugar
- 3 cups water
- 1 cup almond milk
- ¼ cup raisins
- Cinnamon powder to sprinkle

Directions:

At first, take your Instant Pot and one by one add in the mentioned ingredients except almond milk and cinnamon powder. Stir the ingredients well with each other.

Cover and close the pressure vent.

Press "Manual" setting option and set cooking time to 5 minutes. Once the cooking time is done, release the pressure naturally.

Open the lid and stir in the almond milk.

Press "Sauté" and heat the mixture until most of the liquid has evaporated.

Transfer pudding into bowls. Top with the raisins and dash of cinnamon powder; serve warm.

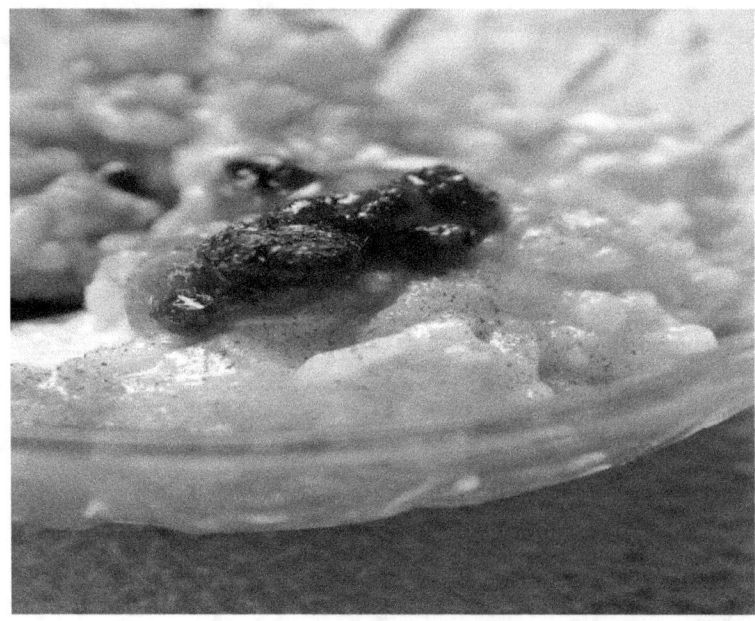

2) Stuffed Apple Treat

Prep Time: 20-25 min.

Serves: 7-8

Approx. Calories (per serving): 341

Ingredients:

- 1/2 cup nut butter, unsweetened
- 2/4 teaspoon nutmeg
- 2 tablespoons almonds or walnuts, finely chopped
- 4 tablespoons cinnamon
- 8 green apples, cored
- 1 cup melted coconut butter
- A large pinch salt
- 1/2 cup coconut, shredded, unsweetened
- 2 cups water

Directions:

In a bowl of medium size, thoroughly mix the coconut butter, nut butter, cinnamon, nutmeg, and salt.

Add this mixture into each apple.

Sprinkle with the shredded coconut. Place the apples in a heatproof bowl and add the bowl over the trivet.

Pour water in the bottom and place the trivet in the Instant Pot. Cover and close the pressure vent.

Press "Slow cook" setting option and set cooking time to 1 hour. Once the cooking time is done, release the pressure naturally. Serve warm.

3) Tangy Berry Delight

Prep Time: 20 min.

Serves: 7-8

Approx. Calories (per serving): 194

Ingredients:

- 4 tablespoons lemon juice
- 2 tablespoons water
- 2 tablespoons cornstarch
- 2 cups blueberries
- 4 cups strawberries, make slices
- 1 1/2 cups sugar

Directions:

Mix the cornstarch with water in a container; set aside.

At first, take your Instant Pot and one by one add the strawberries, sugar, lemon juice and 1/3 of the blueberries. Stir the ingredients well with each other.

Cover and close the pressure vent.

Press "Manual" setting option and set cooking time to 3 minutes. Once the cooking time is done, release the pressure naturally.

Press "Saute" and press "Adjust" setting twice. Add the cornstarch mixture and stir until the mixture thickens.

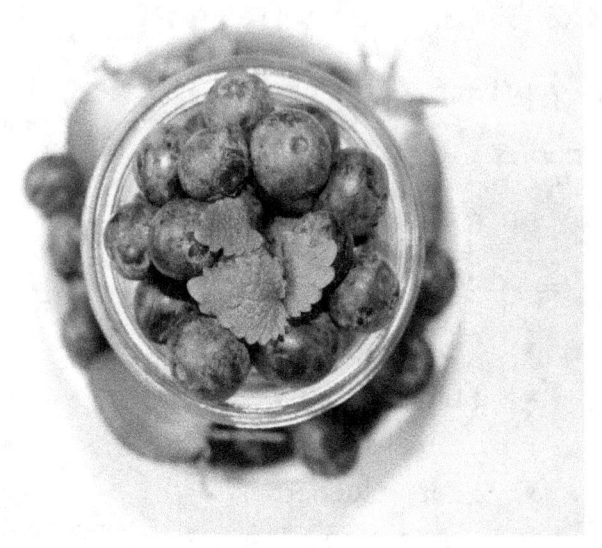

4) Plantains Pineapple Pudding

Prep Time: 25-30 min.

Serves: 4

Approx. Calories (per serving): 247

Ingredients:

- 2 cups ripe pineapple wedges
- 2 cups water
- 2 medium semi ripe plantains, peeled and make halves
- 1 cup brown sugar

Directions:

At first, take your Instant Pot and one by one add in the mentioned ingredients. Stir the ingredients well with each other.

Cover and close the pressure vent.

Press "Manual" setting option and set cooking time to 10 minutes. Once the cooking time is done, release the pressure naturally.

Transfer the pudding into bowls and serve warm.

Store remaining pudding in the fridge for up to one week.

5) Poached Ginger Cinnamon Pears

Prep Time: 25-30 min.

Serves: 4-5

Approx. Calories (per serving): 267

Ingredients:

- 1 cup sugar
- 2 whole cloves
- 1/2 teaspoon cinnamon, ground
- 1/2 teaspoon ginger, minced
- 4 green pears, peeled
- 1 bay leaf
- 3/4 glass of red wine

Directions:

At first, take your Instant Pot and one by one add in the mentioned ingredients except pears. Stir the ingredients well with each other.

Place the pears in the pot, in a standing position.

Cover and close the pressure vent.

Press "Manual" setting option and set cooking time to 8 minutes. Once the cooking time is done, release the pressure naturally.

Place the pears in a serving bowl and discard the leaf.

Press "Saute" and press "Adjust" setting twice. Simmer until the sauce thickens.

Pour the warm sauce over the pears and serve warm.

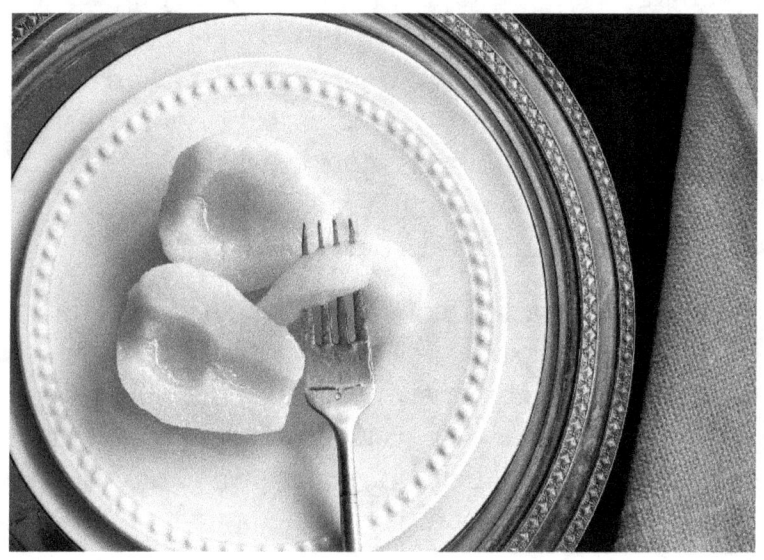

Conclusion

Nothing beats the joy of having a satisfying home-cooked meal at home. With this cookbook, creating delicious and nutritious vegan meals is a breeze as you simply add a few ingredients into your Instant Pot, press a few buttons, and leave the kitchen for some relaxation or family time. When you return, a warm dish is waiting for you.

I sincerely hope this cookbook has succeeded in its aim to help you save time for more important things while using creative ways to make delicious vegan cuisines at home. The versatile recipes covered in this cookbook will help you transform your everyday diet to lead a quality lifestyle.

As always, cooking is an interpretation, so be creative and add your own touch to these recipes to make your customized version and share with your whole family.

Thank you and have a great time enjoying the delicious recipes!

Best of luck in all your endeavors! Happy Cooking!
-- *Lisa Hyde*

P.S. If you enjoyed this dedicated book on Instant Pot Vegan recipes, please take a few minutes of your valuable time to leave a supportive review on Amazon and help make the next version better. Thank you so much!

www.ingramcontent.com/pod-product-compliance
Lightning Source LLC
Chambersburg PA
CBHW071226280526
45787CB00002B/818